PCOS DIET

COOKBOOK

Delicious Recipes For Hormone Balance, Weight Loss, And Insulin Sensitivity

DR ELIAN GRIFFIN

DISCLAIMER

The nutritional recommendations and recipes in this book are meant solely for informative reasons. They are not meant to replace the counsel, diagnosis, or care of a qualified medical expert. If you have any doubts about a medical condition or dietary requirements, you should always see your physician or another trained healthcare expert.

All reasonable efforts have been taken by the author and publisher to ensure that the information contained in this book is correct as of the date of publication. Recommendations may alter, though, as medical knowledge is always changing. When using any of the recipes or instructions found here, the user assumes all liability and assumes no risk, whether personal or otherwise. People who have certain dietary requirements or medical issues should speak with a healthcare provider for personalized guidance. The given recipes are only ideas; you may need to adjust them to suit your own nutritional needs, tastes, and tolerances.

When you use this book, you agree to release the publisher, the author, and their representatives from any liability for any claims, damages, liabilities, costs, or expenditures resulting from your use of the book.

TABLE OF CONTENTS

ABOUT THE BOOK

The "PCOS Diet Cookbook" is an invaluable resource for anyone attempting to navigate the intricacies of Polycystic Ovary Syndrome (PCOS). Understanding the critical role nutrition plays in controlling PCOS symptoms, this cookbook offers a thorough approach to eating healthily while taking into account the special dietary requirements associated with PCOS.

Gaining an understanding of PCOS necessitates first understanding its effects on hormonal balance and metabolic function. This cookbook equips readers with the knowledge necessary to make nutrient-dense, PCOS-friendly dietary choices that can reduce symptoms and promote overall wellness. Every recipe is carefully designed to include important nutrients that are critical for PCOS management, guaranteeing that meals are not only therapeutic but also delicious.

The cookbook starts with foundational knowledge, outlining the fundamentals of nutrition specific to PCOS needs.

It highlights the significance of balanced meals and provides helpful meal planning advice, such as how to read food labels to make the best decisions. With a carefully chosen collection of PCOS-friendly recipes, from hearty breakfasts to filling dinners and healthy snacks, this resource guarantees variety and adequate nutrition.

Cooking techniques like batch cooking and freezer-friendly options help to maintain dietary consistency, which is important when it comes to effectively managing PCOS.

Recipes are created with the preservation of nutrient integrity in mind, using cooking methods that enhance flavors without compromising health goals.

In addition, the cookbook tackles weight management—a problem that many PCOS sufferers face—by including recipes that encourage good eating and exercise regimens. Lifestyle advice highlights stress reduction, good sleep hygiene, and self-care techniques, acknowledging their significant influence on hormone balance and general well-being.

Practical advice guarantees that treating PCOS stays doable and sustainable for people facing social situations or eating out. Frequently asked questions and common concerns are thoroughly addressed, assisting with everything from controlling cravings to seeking expert treatment.

"PCOS Diet Cookbook" is more than just a cookbook; it's a comprehensive resource that gives people the information and skills they need to live a healthy, balanced life while managing PCOS through food and lifestyle choices. Whether you're trying to improve your fertility, lose weight, or just feel better overall, this cookbook is a great resource that's specifically designed with PCOS patients in mind.

CHAPTER ONE

PCOS DIET INTRODUCTION

PCOS DEFINITION

Understanding PCOS entails realizing its impact on hormone regulation and metabolism, which can affect general health and well-being. Polycystic Ovary Syndrome (PCOS) is a common hormonal disorder that affects individuals assigned to females at birth. It is characterized by irregular menstrual cycles, excess androgen levels, and small cysts on the ovaries. It can lead to various symptoms such as infertility, weight gain, acne, and hair growth on the face or body.

A lifestyle that promotes hormone balance and overall health is essential for managing PCOS. This lifestyle includes dietary modifications, consistent exercise, and occasionally medication. By emphasizing nutrition, PCOS sufferers can better control their symptoms and lower their chance of developing long-term health issues.

A balanced diet can help stabilize blood sugar levels, control weight, and reduce inflammation, all of which help manage PCOS symptoms.

DIET IS CRUCIAL FOR MANAGING SYMPTOMS OF PCOS

A PCOS-specific diet typically emphasizes whole foods like fruits, vegetables, lean proteins, and healthy fats while minimizing processed foods, sugars, and refined carbohydrates. This approach helps regulate insulin levels, which is crucial because many PCOS patients are insulin-resistant. Diet plays a pivotal role in managing PCOS symptoms because certain foods can either worsen or alleviate symptoms associated with the condition.

In addition, certain nutrients and supplements such as antioxidants, magnesium, and omega-3 fatty acids may help lower inflammation and support hormone balance. Eating a healthy diet can also help maintain a healthy weight, which can improve fertility outcomes and lower the risk of cardiovascular disease and type 2 diabetes, which are common concerns for those with PCOS.

This PCOS Diet Cookbook offers a variety of tasty and nutritious recipes that are high in fiber, low in refined sugars and carbohydrates, and rich in essential nutrients. All of the recipes are crafted to support hormone balance and promote overall health, making it easier for people with PCOS to maintain a balanced diet without feeling deprived. This cookbook is intended to make meal planning and preparation easier for those who are looking to manage their condition through diet.

You can take charge of your health and well-being by making PCOS-friendly recipes a part of your daily routine.

The cookbook offers helpful advice on how to choose ingredients, portion sizes, and timing of meals to maximize nutrition and effectively manage symptoms. Whether you want to increase fertility, reduce weight, or improve insulin sensitivity, this cookbook is a useful tool for overcoming PCOS's nutritional challenges.

This cookbook contains a wide variety of recipes that can be adjusted to accommodate different dietary requirements and preferences. From filling breakfast options like protein-rich smoothie bowls to satisfying lunch and dinner recipes like vibrant salads, tasty stir-fries, and cozy soups, every dish has been carefully chosen to support your health goals while satisfying your palate. Snacks, desserts, and drinks are also included so that every meal of the day can be enjoyable and nourishing.

Whether you're a cooking novice or an expert, these recipes are made to be accessible and simple to make, with helpful cooking tips and clear instructions provided throughout the cookbook.

The recipes feature ingredients that are known for their beneficial effects on PCOS symptoms, such as leafy greens, lean proteins, nuts, seeds, and whole grains.

To get the most out of this PCOS Diet Cookbook, read through the introduction sections thoroughly to learn about PCOS and what to eat. Make a note of any ingredient substitutions or modifications that are suggested for certain dietary preferences or allergies. Plan your meals by choosing recipes that suit your tastes and nutritional objectives for each meal of the week.

With these tips, you can confidently navigate the cookbook and harness its potential to support your journey toward managing PCOS through balanced nutrition. You can also quickly locate recipes based on ingredients or meal types by using its index and table of contents. It's helpful to plan your grocery shopping around the recipes you intend to prepare, ensuring you have all the necessary ingredients on hand. Try out different recipes to keep your meals interesting and varied while ensuring they support your health objectives.

CHAPTER TWO

KNOWING THE FUNDAMENTALS OF PCOS NUTRITION

Understanding the fundamentals of nutrition is essential to managing PCOS (Polycystic Ovary Syndrome), a condition that affects hormone levels in women of reproductive age. PCOS frequently involves insulin resistance and hormonal imbalances, impacting weight management and fertility. A balanced diet can help regulate these factors. Lean proteins like chicken, fish, and legumes support muscle health and help maintain steady energy levels throughout the day. Healthy fats from sources like nuts, seeds, and avocados provide essential fatty acids necessary for hormone production and absorption of fat-soluble vitamins.

A diet that supports hormone balance stabilizes blood sugar levels, and effectively manages weight is formulated with an understanding of these nutritional principles.

It also ensures a rich supply of vitamins, minerals, and antioxidants, which support immune function and overall health. These fundamental concepts serve as the basis for developing customized nutrition plans that are based on the unique needs of each individual and the symptoms of PCOS, ultimately promoting long-term health and well-being.

THE VALUE OF EATING BALANCED MEALS

Healthy fats, lean proteins, complex carbohydrates, and plenty of fruits and vegetables are the main components of a balanced meal. Complex carbohydrates, which are slowly digested and don't spike blood sugar or insulin-like whole grains, vegetables, and legumes do, are important for managing insulin resistance, a common problem in PCOS. Lean proteins, which include fish, tofu, chicken, turkey, and legumes, provide essential amino acids for muscle maintenance and repair, supporting overall metabolic health.

Balanced meals help people with PCOS maintain stable energy levels, effectively manage weight, and support reproductive health. They also help people absorb fat-soluble vitamins and contribute to hormone production. Nuts, seeds, olive oil, and fatty fish are good sources of healthy fats that aid in the production of hormones and the absorption of fat-soluble vitamins. A variety of colorful fruits and vegetables ensure an intake of essential vitamins, minerals, and antioxidants that are beneficial for overall health and immune function.

ADVICE ON ORGANIZING AND PREPARING MEALS

Incorporating a variety of flavors and textures to keep meals interesting and enjoyable while encouraging adherence to a nutritious diet is one way to effectively plan and prepare meals for PCOS and maintain a healthy diet. Another way to plan is to plan meals to include a variety of foods that support insulin sensitivity and hormone balance.

Finally, batch cooking on the weekends can help prepare meals in advance and ensure that healthy options are easily accessible throughout the week.

Portion control is also important; use smaller plates and utensils to help manage portion sizes and prevent overeating. Lastly, involve family or housemates in meal planning and preparation to foster support and maintain motivation. By putting these tips into practice, people with PCOS can streamline their dietary habits and make healthy eating a sustainable part of their lifestyle. Whole foods should be prioritized when planning, and processed foods that may contain added sugars or unhealthy fats should be minimized.

HOW TO LOOK FOR OPTIONS THAT ARE PCOS-FRIENDLY ON FOOD LABELS

To make well-informed decisions that support PCOS management, you must read food labels. Look at serving sizes to gain an understanding of portion control and calorie intake. Next, look at the total amount of carbohydrates, emphasizing sources of fiber such as whole grains and vegetables that help to stabilize blood sugar levels. Avoid foods high in added sugars because they can exacerbate PCOS symptoms by causing insulin spikes. Finally, look at the types of fats; choose unsaturated fats, such as those found in nuts, seeds, and olive oil, while reducing saturated and trans fats, which can aggravate inflammation and hormonal imbalances.

Furthermore, search for lean protein sources that don't contain unhealthy sugars or additives. Make vitamin and mineral-rich food choices, focusing on items that offer necessary nutrients without being overly caloric or artificial. Watch sodium levels and choose lower-salt options to support heart health and lessen bloating. Finally, give preference to natural, whole ingredients over processed foods with lengthy ingredient lists. Individuals with PCOS who become proficient readers of food labels will be able to make informed decisions about what foods to eat that support hormone balance, weight control, and general health.

OVERVIEW OF ESSENTIAL MINERALS FOR PCOS MANAGEMENT

Essential nutrients are critical for controlling PCOS symptoms and advancing general health.

Pay particular attention to adding nutrients that enhance insulin sensitivity, like magnesium and chromium, which are found in whole grains, nuts, and leafy greens. These minerals help control blood sugar levels, which lowers insulin resistance, which is frequently linked to PCOS. Omega-3 fatty acids, which are abundant in fatty fish like salmon and flaxseeds, have anti-inflammatory qualities that help reduce PCOS symptoms, such as irregular menstruation and acne.

Furthermore, antioxidants such as vitamin E, vitamin C, and selenium, which are present in fruits, vegetables, and nuts, fight oxidative stress and support the reproductive system. Sufficient consumption of these nutrients also boosts immunity and shields cells from damage. It is also important to make sure that you are getting enough iron and vitamin D, as deficiency is common in PCOS women and can aggravate symptoms. Iron-rich foods include lean meats, beans, and fortified cereals; vitamin D is obtained from fatty fish, fortified dairy products, and sunlight exposure.

CHAPTER THREE

LIST OF FOODS SUGGESTED FOR PCOS

A balanced diet high in nutrient-dense foods can be very important in managing PCOS (Polycystic Ovary Syndrome). Whole grains, such as brown rice and quinoa, offer complex carbohydrates for long-term energy and help control blood sugar levels. Lean proteins, like turkey, chicken breast, and tofu, are important for hormone regulation and muscle maintenance. Include lots of fruits and vegetables, especially colorful ones like spinach, berries, and sweet potatoes, which are rich in antioxidants and important vitamins.

Legumes like lentils and chickpeas provide plant-based protein and fiber, which aid in digestion and promote a feeling of fullness. Low-fat dairy or dairy alternatives like almond milk can provide calcium without excess saturated fats.

Healthy fats like avocados, nuts, and olive oil should also be included, as they support hormone production and overall metabolic health.

ADVANTAGES OF EVERY FOOD GROUP

The benefits of each food group that is recommended for PCOS are as follows: lean proteins support muscle health and help keep you feeling fuller for longer, which reduces cravings and supports weight management efforts; fruits and vegetables are rich in vitamins, minerals, and antioxidants that combat inflammation and oxidative stress often associated with PCOS; whole grains provide sustained energy release and help regulate insulin levels, crucial for managing PCOS symptoms like insulin resistance.

Legumes provide a plant-based protein source, helping with muscle maintenance and supporting digestive health with their fiber content. Dairy or dairy alternatives provide calcium and vitamin D, essential for bone health and overall well-being. Healthy fats are essential for hormone balance and support reproductive health. They also contribute to satiety and can help prevent blood sugar spikes.

EXAMPLES OF MEAL PLANS INCLUDING THESE FOODS

A tasty and easy way to create balanced meals for PCOS is to make a Greek yogurt parfait with berries and a sprinkle of nuts for extra protein and healthy fats for breakfast.

A satisfying and nutrient-dense lunch option is a quinoa salad with mixed greens, grilled chicken, avocado, and a light olive oil dressing. For dinner, try baked salmon with roasted sweet potatoes and steamed broccoli, which provides lean protein, healthy fats, lots of fiber, and antioxidants.

Smoothies with spinach, berries, almond milk, and a scoop of protein powder can make a quick and nutrient-dense meal replacement or snack. Other snack options include apple slices with almond butter or a small handful of mixed nuts and seeds for a satisfying and nutrient-dense pick-me-up.

When cooking PCOS-friendly foods, try steaming, baking, grilling, or sautéing them with little to no oil. These cooking techniques hold onto more vitamins and minerals than frying or boiling, which can cause nutrient loss. When cooking veggies, try to achieve bright colors and crunchy textures so they maintain their healthy qualities.

Lean proteins can be marinated or lightly seasoned before cooking to enhance flavor without adding extra calories; substituting herbs and spices for salt can also add flavor and health benefits without compromising nutrient integrity. Grains such as brown rice and quinoa should be cooked as directed by the manufacturer to retain their fiber and nutritional content.

BUYING ADVICE FOR FILLING YOUR PANTRY

To maximize fiber and nutrient intake, choose whole-grain options like quinoa, oats, and whole wheat pasta over refined grains. When stocking your pantry for a PCOS-friendly diet, prioritize fresh produce, lean proteins, whole grains, and healthy fats. When choosing fruits and vegetables, go for fresh or frozen; steer clear of canned varieties that have added sugars or preservatives.

To reduce saturated fat intake while still getting essential nutrients like calcium and vitamin D, choose lean meats like skinless chicken breast or turkey, and think about adding plant-based protein sources like tofu or legumes. To enhance flavor and facilitate cooking, stock up on healthy fats like olive oil, avocados, nuts, and seeds, as well as low-fat dairy options.

CHAPTER FOUR

MEAL PLANNING AND PREPARATION

MEAL PLANNING'S ADVANTAGES FOR PCOS MANAGEMENT

Planning meals ahead of time allows people with PCOS to make sure they are consuming the right balance of nutrients, such as lean proteins, complex carbohydrates, and healthy fats. It also helps to avoid processed foods and excessive sugars, which can exacerbate insulin resistance—a common issue in PCOS. Finally, meal planning gives people with PCOS less stress when it comes to deciding what to eat each day, which makes it easier to stick to a healthy eating routine.

Additionally, meal planning can help people reach and maintain a healthy weight, which is crucial for managing PCOS. By planning for portion sizes and nutritional value, people can avoid overindulging and keep their blood sugar levels stable throughout the day, which can help lessen cravings and mood swings that are frequently linked to PCOS. In summary, the methodical process of meal planning not only benefits physical health but also fosters emotional well-being by lowering anxiety related to food choices.

HOW TO MAKE A MEAL PLAN THAT IS PCOS-FRIENDLY

A PCOS-friendly meal plan should emphasize nutrient-dense foods that support insulin sensitivity and hormone balance. To start, include lots of vitamin, mineral, and fiber-rich non-starchy vegetables (think leafy greens, broccoli, and peppers); lean proteins (think chicken, fish, tofu, or legumes) to help stabilize blood sugar levels and promote satiety; and complex carbohydrates (think quinoa, sweet potatoes, and whole grains) that digest more slowly and prevent blood sugar spikes.

Aim for balanced meals that include a combination of protein, healthy fats, and carbohydrates to support overall health and well-being. It's also beneficial to incorporate PCOS-specific superfoods like berries, nuts, seeds, and omega-3 fatty acids found in fish or flaxseed oil, which can help reduce inflammation and improve insulin sensitivity. When planning meals, think about spacing them evenly throughout the day to maintain steady energy levels and prevent excessive hunger.

COOKING IN BULK AND FREEZER-FRIENDLY RECIPES

Batch cooking is a time-saving technique that involves making large batches of meals ahead of time and freezing them for later use. This works especially well for people with PCOS because it guarantees that they will always have access to homemade, healthful meals, even on hectic days. Look for recipes that are simple to scale up, like casseroles, stews, soups, and stir-fries, which can be portioned and frozen for ease of use. Label and date each meal to monitor freshness and guarantee variety in your weekly diet.

By preserving leftovers or excess portions, freezer-friendly meals allow for flexibility and reduce food waste. When batch cooking, use freezer-safe containers or zip-top bags to store individual servings that can be thawed and reheated as needed.

This method not only saves time but also promotes mindful eating habits by avoiding impulsive food choices. People with PCOS can maintain a consistent and nourishing diet without the hassle of preparing meals every day.

ADVICE FOR ORGANIZING MEALS EFFECTIVELY WITH PCOS-FRIENDLY RECIPES

Strategic planning and organization are the first steps toward effective meal prep. Choose recipes that support PCOS dietary guidelines, emphasizing whole foods and balanced nutrition. Prepare ingredients ahead of time by washing and chopping vegetables, marinating proteins, and cooking grains. Use portion control tools, such as measuring cups, scales, and meal prep containers, to ensure balanced servings that support blood sugar control and weight management.

Meal prep can be made more efficient by designating a specific day of the week and allocating a specific amount of time to prepare meals. To stay organized and monitor your progress, make a meal prep schedule or checklist. Try different cooking techniques, like baking, roasting, steaming, or sautéing, to add variety to your meals while maintaining vital nutrients. By implementing these strategies, people with PCOS can make meal preparation easier, save time, and prioritize their health by maintaining consistent, nutrient-dense eating habits.

RESOURCES AND TOOLS FOR EFFECTIVE MEAL PLANNING

Start by using meal planning apps or websites that offer customizable templates, recipe databases, and grocery list features tailored to PCOS-friendly diets. These tools can help streamline the planning process by suggesting nutrient-dense recipes and calculating serving sizes based on individual dietary needs. Successful meal planning for PCOS requires access to trustworthy tools and resources that support dietary goals and lifestyle preferences.

Purchase high-quality kitchen necessities like sharp knives, chopping boards, food storage bins, and cooking utensils to make meal preparation more efficient.

A slow cooker or instant pot can be purchased for easy one-pot meals that require little work and produce a lot of flavor. Fill your pantry with staples like whole grains, canned beans, spices, and herbs to make meals taste better and be more nutritious without adding sugar or preservatives.

Moreover, look for assistance from online forums, communities, or social media groups devoted to PCOS nutrition and meal planning. Interacting with people who have comparable health objectives can inspire you, offer recipe suggestions, and offer useful advice on how to keep a balanced diet. By employing these tools and resources, PCOS sufferers can take charge of their nutrition, enhance their general health, and develop long-lasting meal-planning habits.

THE VALUE OF A BALANCED BREAKFAST IN THE MANAGEMENT OF PCOS

Incorporating complex carbohydrates, lean proteins, and healthy fats into your morning meal helps prevent blood sugar spikes and promotes better hormone balance throughout the day. This approach not only supports weight management but also helps reduce symptoms like irregular periods and unwanted hair growth associated with PCOS. Eating a balanced breakfast is essential for managing PCOS effectively, especially for women who often experience insulin resistance.

A healthy breakfast also speeds up your metabolism, which can help with weight management—a common issue for women with PCOS. You can give your body sustained energy by eschewing sugary cereals and pastries in favor of whole grains, fresh fruits, and protein-rich foods like eggs or Greek yogurt. Because of hormonal fluctuations, PCOS patients often struggle to focus and be productive throughout the morning. You can also reduce bloating and discomfort by including foods high in fiber, which helps regulate digestion.

Overall, starting your day with a nutritious breakfast sets a positive tone for managing PCOS symptoms and promoting overall health. Additionally, a well-rounded breakfast can support emotional well-being by stabilizing mood swings and reducing cravings for unhealthy snacks later in the day. This is especially important for managing PCOS symptoms like mood swings and emotional eating tendencies.

SIMPLE AND FAST BREAKFAST RECIPES

Easy breakfast recipes can help you maintain a healthy diet when managing PCOS. Look for recipes that can be put together in a matter of minutes, like yogurt parfaits with layered fruits and nuts, or overnight oats. These recipes not only save time but also guarantee that you get a good balance of the proteins, fats, and carbohydrates that are necessary for managing PCOS symptoms.

Rich in nutrients and a good source of protein that helps stabilize blood sugar levels and supports hormone balance throughout the day, a vegetable omelet made with spinach, tomatoes, and a sprinkle of cheese is another fantastic option. Smoothies filled with leafy greens, berries, and a protein source like Greek yogurt or protein powder are also quick and easy breakfast options that can be enjoyed on the go.

Whole grain pancakes or waffles with Greek yogurt and fresh fruit on top can satiate sweet tooths while supplying vital nutrients. These breakfast options are adaptable and can be tailored to individual preferences and dietary requirements, which makes them perfect for effectively managing PCOS symptoms.

RICH IN NUTRIENT SMOOTHIES AND SHAKES

Smoothies and shakes are a great option for women with PCOS because they can be made with nutrient-dense ingredients that support hormone balance and general health. Add fruits like berries, which are low in sugar but high in antioxidants and fiber, which help control blood sugar levels, to a base of leafy greens like spinach or kale, which are rich in folate and other essential vitamins.

Protein is essential for controlling PCOS symptoms because it helps stabilize blood sugar levels and supports muscle health. Healthy fats like avocado or nut butter can further improve the nutritional profile of your smoothie by offering sustained energy and promoting satiety. To boost protein intake, include ingredients like Greek yogurt, almond milk, or protein powder made from sources like peas or collagen.

Experiment with different flavor combinations and textures to keep your smoothies exciting and enjoyable while supporting your PCOS management goals. Superfoods, such as chia seeds or flaxseeds, are rich in omega-3 fatty acids and fiber and can help regulate hormone levels and reduce inflammation, which is beneficial for women with PCOS. Furthermore, these ingredients support heart health.

Using whole grains like quinoa or oats instead of refined grains can help stabilize blood sugar levels and increase fiber intake. These grains can be cooked into porridges or used as a base for breakfast bowls topped with nuts, seeds, and fresh fruit. Creating a creative and delicious breakfast can be a great way to incorporate PCOS-friendly ingredients into your diet.

To make sure you consume enough protein without going overboard with saturated fats, opt for lean proteins like eggs, tofu, or lean meats. Eggs can be blended into smoothies or stir-fried with vegetables for a satisfying breakfast option. Eggs can also be baked into muffin tin omelets or scrambled with vegetables.

Nut butter can be spread on whole-grain toast or mixed into oatmeal for added flavor and nutritional benefits. Avocado toast topped with a poached egg and a sprinkle of chia seeds is a nutrient-dense and satisfying breakfast option.

Healthy fats like avocados, nuts, and seeds can be incorporated into your breakfast recipes to support hormone balance and promote satiety.

When managing PCOS symptoms, meal prep can save your sanity on hectic mornings. Take some time on the weekends or in the evenings to prepare breakfast ingredients that you can quickly assemble or reheat during the week. Make a big batch of overnight oats or chia seed pudding and portion them into individual containers for breakfasts that you can grab on the go.

Smoothie packs can be made by portioning fruits, greens, and protein sources ahead of time and freezing them.

Then, in the morning, just add your preferred liquid base and blend for a wholesome breakfast in a matter of minutes. Vegetable and cheese egg muffins can be baked in advance, frozen, and then reheated for a quick and high-protein breakfast option.

If you're looking for a quick and simple breakfast that can be customized with toppings like yogurt and fresh berries, try batch-cooking whole-grain pancakes or waffles and freezing them in single portions. Having pre-cut fruits and vegetables on hand also makes it easier to add nutritious sides to your breakfast, ensuring you get a variety of vitamins and minerals to support overall health and PCOS management.

By putting these meal prep suggestions into practice, you can simplify your morning routine and make sure you always have wholesome breakfast options on hand. This will set the stage for a well-balanced diet that will effectively support PCOS management.

For example, a quinoa salad with grilled chicken, mixed greens, and a variety of colorful vegetables offers a satisfying blend of nutrients. Alternatively, a whole-grain wrap filled with hummus, roasted vegetables, and avocado offers a fiber-rich option that promotes satiety. While managing PCOS, maintaining stable energy levels throughout the day is crucial. Making nutritious lunch choices can help stabilize blood sugar levels and support overall well-being.

An additional suggestion would be to make a thick soup of vegetables enhanced with legumes, such as lentils or chickpeas, to add extra protein and fiber. Serve this with a side of whole-grain bread to round out the meal. These lunch options not only boost energy levels but also offer vital nutrients that help control PCOS symptoms. By emphasizing healthy ingredients and well-balanced nutrition, you can make lunches that sustain your energy levels and leave you feeling full and energized all day.

CUSTOMIZED SOUPS, SALADS, AND WRAPS FOR PCOS

You can customize salads, wraps, and soups to fit a PCOS-friendly diet. For a satisfying meal, use whole-grain tortillas filled with lean meats or plant-based proteins, lots of fresh vegetables, and a smear of avocado for healthy fats. Start with a nutrient-rich salad made of leafy greens like spinach or kale, topped with lean protein like grilled salmon or tofu.

Add a variety of colorful vegetables like bell peppers, tomatoes, and cucumbers for extra vitamins and minerals.

Salads, wraps, and soups can be tasty and supportive additions to your PCOS diet by emphasizing whole foods and minimizing processed ingredients. Make a vegetable-rich broth and add beans or lentils for protein. Add whole grains like barley or quinoa for extra fiber and complex carbohydrates.

These soups not only nourish but also provide a low-calorie, high-nutrient meal option ideal for managing PCOS symptoms.

METHODS FOR PUTTING TOGETHER A PCOS-FRIENDLY LUNCH

Making a PCOS-friendly lunch can be easy with a little planning. To guarantee that you have wholesome options on hand, start by making meals in advance. Choose reusable containers that keep food fresh and are convenient to carry. You can also batch-cook items like quinoa, grilled chicken breast, or roasted vegetables to use in multiple meals throughout the week. This method saves time and guarantees that you have a variety of balanced meals available.

Packing lunches this way not only supports your nutritional needs but also helps regulate blood sugar levels, which is beneficial for effectively managing PCOS symptoms. Aim for a mix of lean proteins, such as fish, poultry, or legumes, combined with complex carbohydrates like whole grains or sweet potatoes.

Incorporate plenty of colorful vegetables to provide essential vitamins, minerals, and fiber.

RECIPES FOR HEALTHY LUNCHES THAT ARE STILL SATISFYING

To make satisfying midday meals while controlling PCOS, look for recipes that emphasize flavor and nutrient density. For example, make a grain bowl with quinoa, chickpeas, roasted vegetables, and a drizzle of olive oil for a Mediterranean-inspired meal that provides a good balance of fiber, protein, and healthy fats. Another great option is a salad that is high in protein and consists of mixed greens, grilled chicken or tofu, nuts or seeds, and a light vinaigrette dressing.

Try a whole-grain wrap with hummus, fresh veggies, and lean protein like grilled tempeh or turkey for a heartier meal. These recipes support your dietary goals for managing PCOS while offering variety and flavor. By emphasizing wholesome ingredients and thoughtful portion sizes, you can make midday meals that satiate hunger and enhance overall well-being.

Making educated decisions to support your health goals when navigating restaurant menus and managing PCOS is necessary. Seek out restaurants that provide customizable options, like changing side dishes to steamed vegetables or a side salad; choose grilled, baked, or steamed protein sources, like fish, chicken, or tofu, rather than fried or breaded options; select meals that have an abundance of vegetables and whole grains; and request dressings or sauces on the side to keep portions and ingredients under control.

Preparing ahead of time and making thoughtful decisions will help you enjoy dining out while managing PCOS effectively. Keep in mind that moderation and balance are key to maintaining a PCOS-friendly diet even when dining away from home. When dining out, prioritize balanced meals that include lean proteins, fiber-rich carbohydrates, and healthy fats.

HEALTHY DINNER RECIPES TO HELP CONTROL PCOS SYMPTOMS

Developing dinner recipes that are balanced and help manage PCOS symptoms involves emphasizing foods that are high in nutrients and that help balance hormones and blood sugar.

Lean proteins, like fish, turkey, or chicken breast, provide essential amino acids without being overly saturated. These proteins are best paired with complex carbohydrates, like quinoa, brown rice, or sweet potatoes, to encourage a steady release of energy and avoid insulin spikes.

A significant portion of your meal should consist of vegetables, which provide fiber, vitamins, and minerals that are essential for general health. Choose vibrant vegetables such as bell peppers, broccoli, and leafy greens, as they are high in antioxidants and can help reduce inflammation that is frequently linked to PCOS.

Include healthy fats from nuts, avocado, or olive oil to promote hormone production and the absorption of fat-soluble vitamins.

Balanced dinner recipes can be anything from a stir-fry of lean protein, mixed vegetables, and a light soy sauce or citrus-based dressing to grilled salmon with quinoa and roasted vegetables. These meals are satisfying and support your PCOS management goals while providing essential nutrients, variety, and flavor.

SHEET PAN DINNERS AND ONE-POT MEALS

One-pot meals, such as quinoa and vegetable stews or hearty soups with beans and lean meats, allow for easy preparation and cooking in one pot. These dishes often include a combination of protein, complex carbohydrates, and vegetables, offering a complete and balanced meal in one serving. Sheet pan dinners and one-pot meals are convenient options that minimize cleanup while maximizing nutrition for busy individuals managing PCOS.

Cooking is made even easier with sheet pan dinners, which let you roast a variety of ingredients on one baking sheet. For instance, you can roast chicken thighs with root vegetables, such as carrots and potatoes, seasoned with some olive oil and herbs. This cooking technique enhances flavors and retains nutrients without using a lot of extra fats or sauces.

One-pot dishes and sheet pan dinners can be tailored to feature PCOS-friendly components like lean proteins, whole grains, and an abundance of vibrant vegetables; they are adaptable enough to suit a variety of dietary needs and can be made in advance for easy reheating on hectic evenings.

PLANT-BASED DINNER OPTIONS THAT ARE PCOS-FRIENDLY

Incorporating plant-based options into your dinner routine involves focusing on whole foods like legumes, tofu, tempeh, and a variety of vegetables. These ingredients provide fiber, vitamins, minerals, and phytonutrients essential for hormonal balance and overall health. Plant-based diets can be highly beneficial for managing PCOS symptoms by reducing inflammation and improving insulin sensitivity.

Think of meals like stuffed peppers with black beans and quinoa, stir-fried tofu with mixed vegetables and sesame ginger sauce, or lentil and vegetable curry. These plant-based dinners are not only filling but also tasty, providing a variety of flavors and textures to keep meals interesting.

A well-rounded and satisfying meal that supports your PCOS management goals can be achieved by adding sources of healthy fats, such as nuts, seeds, avocado, and olive oil, to plant-based dinners. These fats support hormone production and the absorption of fat-soluble vitamins.

COOKING METHODS THAT INCORPORATE FLAVOR WITHOUT ENDANGERING HEALTH

For delicious and PCOS-friendly dinners, it's important to use cooking methods that enhance flavor without sacrificing health. For example, use low-oil grilling, roasting, steaming, or sautéing to preserve nutrients and bring out the natural flavors of your ingredients. This way, ingredients can develop caramelization and depth of flavor without needing excess fats or sugars.

You can flavor and tenderize the texture of proteins like chicken, fish, or tofu by marinating them in herbs, spices, and citrus juices before cooking. This way adds flavor without adding extra salt or calorie-dense sauces. Try experimenting with fresh herbs, garlic, ginger, and spicy spices like turmeric, cumin, and paprika to make dishes that are bright and filling.

To enhance savory flavors naturally, add umami-rich ingredients like tomatoes, mushrooms, miso paste, or nutritional yeast. These ingredients can improve the taste profile of your meals and offer extra nutritional value. By learning these cooking techniques, you can make delicious meals that will help you on your PCOS management journey.

Prioritize well-balanced meals that satisfy different palates and dietary requirements when creating family-friendly dinner ideas that are also PCOS-friendly. Begin with tried-and-true favorites like quinoa pilaf and grilled chicken with a side of roasted vegetables, making sure that each ingredient has nutritional benefits that are appropriate for controlling PCOS symptoms. Add a range of tastes and textures to make meals fun for everyone at the table.

Make meals that are adaptable, such as taco nights with whole-grain tortillas, lean ground turkey or beans, and a variety of toppings like avocado, salsa, and shredded lettuce. This way, everyone in the family can put together a plate that suits their tastes while still getting a balanced diet.

On pasta nights, go for whole-grain or legume-based pasta with a homemade marinara sauce that's bursting with veggies like bell peppers, spinach, and zucchini. To increase the meal's nutritional value and satiety, toss in some lean proteins like grilled shrimp or chicken. These dinner ideas are great for the whole family and encourage eating well while taking into account the dietary restrictions associated with PCOS management.

With a little creativity and some tasty dinner ideas, you can plan nutritious meals that will suit the needs of the whole family and help you achieve your PCOS control goals.

THE VALUE OF NUTRITIOUS SNACKS FOR PCOS MANAGEMENT

Choosing nutrient-dense snacks can help prevent spikes in insulin levels, which is beneficial for women with PCOS who often struggle with insulin resistance. These snacks should ideally be balanced with a combination of protein, healthy fats, and complex carbohydrates to promote satiety and prevent sudden drops in blood sugar that can lead to cravings and energy crashes. Snacking healthily is important for managing PCOS (Polycystic Ovary Syndrome) because it helps stabilize blood sugar levels and manage weight, both of which are important factors in PCOS management.

Including healthy snacks in your diet at various times of the day can also help control your appetite and lessen the chance that you will overeat during your main meals. This strategy can help you maintain a stable energy level, which can help with weight management and reduce symptoms like fatigue and mood swings that are often associated with PCOS. Choosing snacks that are high in fiber, vitamins, and minerals, like fruits, vegetables, nuts, and whole grains, can provide vital nutrients that support overall health and hormone balance in women with PCOS.

Women with PCOS can take charge of their nutrition and enhance their general health by making educated snack choices. By emphasizing nutrient-dense foods and steering clear of processed foods heavy in sugar and bad fats, people with PCOS can better control their symptoms and enhance their quality of life.

EASY SNACK RECIPES FOR TRAVEL

For busy women with PCOS, finding quick, portable, and healthy snack ideas is crucial to sustaining energy levels throughout the day without turning to unhealthy options. For example, fresh fruit combined with a small amount of nuts or seeds offers a balanced combination of carbohydrates, protein, and healthy fats; Greek yogurt with berries and granola sprinkled on top offers a satisfying blend of fiber and protein.

Smoothies made with spinach, berries, and a protein source like almond butter or protein powder can be prepared ahead of time and taken on the go for a quick and nutritious snack option.

Hard-boiled eggs are another excellent choice, offering protein and essential nutrients in a portable package. Hummus with carrot or cucumber sticks offers a crunchy, satisfying snack rich in fiber and vitamins.

Women with PCOS can successfully control their hunger and sustain steady energy levels throughout the day by making a plan ahead of time and having these easy-to-make but nourishing snack options in mind.

HEALTHY SWEETS TO SATISFY CRAVINGS

For women with PCOS, controlling cravings is a common challenge, but selecting nutrient-dense treats can help satisfy cravings without compromising health goals. Selecting snacks that combine heart-healthy fats, protein, and fiber can promote satiety and lessen the urge to overindulge in less nutritious options.

Three examples of such snacks are avocado slices drizzled with olive oil and topped with a sprinkle of sea salt.

Chia seed pudding made with almond milk and topped with berries is another nutrient-dense treat rich in fiber, omega-3 fatty acids, and antioxidants. Dark chocolate with a high cocoa content (70% or higher) can satisfy a sweet tooth while providing antioxidants and a modest amount of sugar. Cottage cheese with fresh fruit or whole grain crackers offers a satisfying blend of protein and carbohydrates that can curb cravings and provide sustained energy.

Women with PCOS can have filling snacks that promote their general health and well-being by including these nutrient-dense delights in their diet.

RECIPES FOR DESSERTS AND SNACKS MADE AT HOME

Making homemade snacks and desserts gives PCOS women the ability to maintain control over the ingredients and make sure they meet their specific dietary needs and health objectives. Easy recipes such as oat-nut-butter energy balls provide a healthy snack full of fiber, protein, and healthy fats. Cinnamon-sprinkled baked sweet potato fries satisfy cravings for a sweet and savory treat while providing fiber and vitamin A.

For dessert, a homemade Greek yogurt parfait with layers of yogurt, fresh berries, and granola or nuts can satiate sweet tooths while providing a healthy dose of protein and carbohydrates. Smoothie bowls with frozen fruit blends, spinach, and protein powder make for a nutrient-dense, reviving option that can be personalized with different toppings like chia seeds or coconut flakes.

Women with PCOS can support their health and fitness objectives by experimenting with homemade snacks and desserts and enjoying delectable treats while making thoughtful ingredient and quantity control choices.

TIPS ON PORTION CONTROL FOR PCOS SNACKING

To prevent overeating and maintain a healthy balance of nutrients, women with PCOS must practice portion control. Using smaller bowls or plates for snacks can visually reduce portion sizes and prevent overeating. Measuring snacks is important to prevent overconsumption.

Additionally, choosing snacks that come in single-serving packages or dividing larger portions into smaller servings can support portion control goals. Pre-portioning snacks into individual servings, such as packing nuts or trail mix into small containers, can help avoid mindless eating and promote mindful snacking habits.

By practicing portion control and mindful eating, women with PCOS can better manage their symptoms and support their overall health goals. Being aware of hunger cues and eating slowly can further help women with PCOS listen to their bodies and recognize when they are truly hungry versus eating out of habit or emotion.

CHAPTER FIVE

PCOS AND CONTROLLING WEIGHT

RECOGNIZING THE CONNECTION BETWEEN PCOS AND WEIGHT

Weight gain, especially around the abdomen, is a common symptom of Polycystic Ovary Syndrome (PCOS), which is characterized by hormonal imbalances that affect metabolism and insulin sensitivity. Insulin resistance, a common feature of PCOS, leads to increased production of insulin by the pancreas, which in turn promotes fat storage and makes weight loss more difficult. It is important to understand this link to develop effective strategies to manage weight with PCOS.

Focusing on dietary modifications is essential to addressing the weight implications of PCOS. Regular physical activity is essential for managing weight and improving insulin sensitivity. Strength training and aerobic exercises are especially helpful for burning calories and increasing muscle mass, which can help regulate metabolism and support weight loss goals. A diet low in refined carbohydrates and sugars can help manage insulin levels and support weight loss efforts. Lean proteins, whole grains, and plenty of vegetables can stabilize blood sugar levels and reduce the risk of insulin spikes that contribute to weight gain.

TECHNIQUES FOR PCOS PATIENTS TO MANAGE THEIR WEIGHT HEALTHILY

A combination of dietary adjustments, consistent exercise, and lifestyle changes is necessary for effective weight management with PCOS. A low-glycemic index (GI) diet, which emphasizes foods that release sugar slowly into the bloodstream, can help stabilize insulin levels and manage weight. It is important to emphasize foods like whole grains, legumes, lean proteins, and healthy fats while limiting processed foods and sugary snacks. This dietary approach not only supports weight loss but also enhances general health and lowers the risk of PCOS-related complications.

Apart from diet, regular physical activity is essential for managing weight with PCOS. 150 minutes a week of moderate-intensity exercise, like brisk walking, swimming, or cycling, burns calories, improves insulin sensitivity, and aids in weight loss. Strength training exercises, like lifting weights or using resistance bands, can also increase muscle mass and metabolism, which further aids in weight management. Maintaining a healthy body weight with PCOS requires consistency and adherence to these lifestyle changes.

TIPS FOR EXERCISE TO GO ALONG WITH YOUR DIET

Incorporating both aerobic and strength training exercises into your routine is essential. Aerobic exercises, such as jogging, dancing, or aerobics classes, help burn calories and improve cardiovascular fitness. Aim for at least 30 minutes of moderate-intensity aerobic activity most days of the week to maximize benefits. Exercise is a cornerstone of managing weight with PCOS, helping to burn calories, improve insulin sensitivity, and support overall health.

Weightlifting, resistance band exercises, and bodyweight exercises like lunges and squats are examples of strength-training activities that contribute to the development of lean muscle mass. Since muscle burns more calories than fat, increasing muscle mass through strength training can increase metabolism and help with weight management. Try to incorporate strength training activities into your routine at least twice or three times a week, focusing on your major muscle groups for best results.

RECIPES DEVELOPED TO ASSIST IN LOSING WEIGHT

Meal planning for PCOS-accounting weight loss involves selecting nutrient-dense foods that lower insulin resistance and support stable blood sugar levels; lean proteins (like turkey, chicken, or tofu) that provide energy and fiber without raising blood sugar levels; and whole grains (like quinoa, brown rice, or oats) that satisfy hunger and support muscle maintenance.

An important component of PCOS-friendly meals should be vegetables, which provide vitamins, minerals, and antioxidants that promote overall health. Leafy greens, broccoli, bell peppers, and spinach are great options for salads, stir-fries, or soups. Healthy fats from sources like avocados, nuts, and olive oil offer essential fatty acids and help you feel full and satisfied.

When cooking, pay attention to portion sizes that are balanced and include protein, healthy fats, and carbohydrates high in fiber to support weight loss goals and effectively manage PCOS symptoms.

MONITORING DEVELOPMENT AND CREATING PRACTICAL OBJECTIVES

Keep a food diary to record meals, snacks, and portion sizes along with any symptoms or changes in weight. This helps identify patterns and make necessary changes to your diet and exercise routine. Tracking food intake, physical activity, and weight changes can provide valuable insights into what works best for your body. Monitoring progress and setting realistic goals are essential for long-term success in managing weight with PCOS.

Achieving small, attainable goals like increasing daily physical activity, cutting back on sugary snacks, or adding more vegetables to meals will help you stay motivated and make progress. Celebrate small victories along the way, like hitting a milestone in your weight loss journey or sticking to your exercise schedule. As you make progress, adjust your goals to keep pushing yourself and to keep making positive changes in managing your weight with PCOS.

CHAPTER SIX

LIFESTYLE SUGGESTIONS FOR PCOS WELLBEING

MODIFYING ONE'S LIFESTYLE IS CRUCIAL FOR MANAGING PCOS

A balanced diet that supports hormone regulation and insulin sensitivity is one of the most important ways to manage PCOS (polycystic ovary syndrome). PCOS-friendly diets typically consist of whole foods like fruits, vegetables, lean proteins, and healthy fats, while minimizing processed foods and sugars. This helps to stabilize blood sugar levels and reduce insulin resistance, which are common issues in PCOS.

Regular physical activity is also important because it helps to maintain a healthy weight, improve insulin sensitivity, and reduce stress levels—all of which contribute to the effective management of PCOS symptoms. Even moderate exercise, like yoga or brisk walking, can have positive effects.

For women with PCOS, stress management is just as important as diet and exercise. Stress increases cortisol levels and upsets hormonal balance, which exacerbates symptoms. Mindfulness meditation, deep breathing exercises, and yoga are some of the techniques that help reduce stress and promote relaxation. These practices not only improve mental health but also support overall hormone regulation and PCOS symptom management. Including these lifestyle changes in your daily routine can result in noticeable improvements in PCOS symptoms as well as overall quality of life.

Education regarding PCOS and its management is also essential. By comprehending how lifestyle factors impact symptoms and making the necessary adjustments, people can take charge of their health. It's also critical to seek the advice of medical professionals who specialize in PCOS management, such as nutritionists and endocrinologists. These professionals can offer individualized guidance and support that is tailored to each patient's needs, ensuring a successful approach to managing this complex condition.

THE EFFECTS OF STRESS MANAGEMENT STRATEGIES ON PCOS

Developing a regular stress management routine can greatly improve the overall health and quality of life of women with PCOS. Stress management is essential for effectively managing the symptoms of PCOS because chronic stress can exacerbate insulin resistance and hormonal imbalances, which are the core issues in PCOS. Stress management techniques like progressive muscle relaxation, journaling, and mindfulness meditation can help reduce stress and promote emotional well-being.

These practices also help to lower cortisol levels, which in turn support hormone balance and alleviate symptoms like acne and irregular periods.

Apart from relaxation techniques, regular physical activity can also help reduce stress. Exercise releases endorphins, which are naturally occurring mood enhancers, and can enhance sleep quality. This twofold benefit not only helps reduce stress but also supports hormone regulation and weight management, two crucial aspects of managing PCOS. You can make exercise a sustainable part of your lifestyle by finding activities you enjoy, like dancing, swimming, or even gardening.

By prioritizing stress management and seeking support, women with PCOS can take proactive steps toward improving their overall well-being. Creating a strong support network is equally important to effectively managing stress and PCOS. Reaching out to others who understand your experiences, whether through support groups or online forums, can offer emotional support and useful advice. Sharing experiences and tips for managing stress and PCOS symptoms can be empowering and help in navigating the challenges of living with this condition.

TIPS FOR GOOD SLEEP HYGIENE FOR HORMONE BALANCE

Women with PCOS need to practice good sleep hygiene because getting enough sleep is essential for hormone balance and general health. Regular sleep schedules, like going to bed and waking up at the same time every day, help regulate circadian rhythms and promote restorative sleep. Having a soothing bedtime routine, like taking a warm bath or using relaxation techniques, helps the body wind down and fall asleep more easily. Reducing stimulants, like caffeine and electronics, before bed can further improve the quality of sleep.

Establishing a comfortable sleeping environment is also crucial. To ensure uninterrupted sleep, keep your bedroom cool, dark, and quiet. Invest in a supportive mattress and pillows that meet your comfort preferences. Before bed, try mindfulness or gentle yoga to help calm your mind and relax your body, setting the stage for a restful night's sleep. For women with PCOS, prioritizing sleep hygiene practices can have a significant impact on hormone regulation and overall well-being.

Women with PCOS can optimize their health and well-being by prioritizing sleep hygiene practices and seeking appropriate support if sleep disturbances persist despite following good sleep hygiene. Sleep disorders, such as sleep apnea, are more common in PCOS women and can contribute to hormonal imbalances and other health issues.

Addressing sleep concerns with a healthcare provider can lead to personalized recommendations or treatments that improve sleep quality and support overall PCOS management.

INCLUDING SELF-CARE PRACTICES IN YOUR EVERYDAY LIFE

Self-care involves activities that promote physical, emotional, and mental health, helping to reduce stress and support hormone balance. Making time each day for self-care activities like meditation, gentle exercise, or enjoyable hobbies can help you feel refreshed and relaxed. These practices also help manage PCOS symptoms like mood swings and irregular periods by lowering cortisol levels and promoting emotional resilience.

Women with PCOS must incorporate self-care routines into their daily lives to effectively manage their symptoms and improve their overall well-being.

Planning and prepping meals ahead of time can make it easier to maintain a nutritious diet amidst a busy schedule, ensuring consistent energy levels and overall well-being. Nutrition also plays a significant role in self-care for women with PCOS.

Adopting a balanced diet rich in whole foods such as fruits, vegetables, lean proteins, and healthy fats supports hormone regulation and insulin sensitivity. Avoiding processed foods and sugars can help stabilize blood sugar levels and reduce inflammation, which is beneficial for managing PCOS symptoms.

Building a strong support network enables sharing experiences and coping strategies related to living with PCOS, fostering a sense of belonging and understanding. Furthermore, in addition to physical and dietary practices, nurturing social connections is important for self-care.

Women with PCOS can improve their quality of life and effectively manage their health by prioritizing self-care and incorporating these practices into their daily lives. Spending time with supportive friends and family members, or participating in community activities, can provide emotional support and reduce feelings of isolation.

SOURCES OF ADDITIONAL INFORMATION AND SUPPORT

For women with PCOS who want to learn more about their condition and effectively manage its symptoms, it is important to find trustworthy resources for additional support and information.

Medical professionals, including gynecologists, endocrinologists, and registered dietitians with expertise in PCOS management, can offer individualized guidance and treatment options, as well as insights into hormonal imbalances, insulin resistance, and lifestyle modifications that are customized to each patient's needs. Consultations with healthcare providers regularly ensure ongoing support and necessary modifications to treatment plans.

Engaging with online resources can help women with PCOS make informed decisions about their health and well-being. Websites, forums, and social media groups offer opportunities to connect with others who have experienced similar things, offering emotional support and useful advice.

These platforms frequently feature articles, podcasts, and webinars hosted by healthcare experts and advocates, covering topics like nutrition, fitness, mental health, and fertility-related to PCOS.

A combination of professional advice, community support, and educational materials empowers women with PCOS to take proactive steps toward improving their quality of life. Educational materials such as books, articles, and research studies on PCOS offer thorough insights into the condition's causes, symptoms, and treatment options.

These resources aid in understanding the underlying mechanisms of PCOS and the significance of lifestyle changes in effectively managing symptoms.

Women who are well-informed about the most recent advancements in PCOS research and treatment can take charge of their health and work with healthcare providers to optimize their care.

CHAPTER SEVEN

ANSWERING FREQUENTLY ASKED QUESTIONS ABOUT DIET AND PCOS

A balanced diet rich in whole foods, lean proteins, healthy fats, and complex carbohydrates is generally recommended. This helps regulate insulin levels, which is important as insulin resistance is common in PCOS. Additionally, focusing on low glycemic index foods can help stabilize blood sugar levels and reduce inflammation associated with PCOS. Many women with PCOS wonder what type of diet is best for them.

It's also typical to wonder how certain diets, such as low-carb or ketogenic diets, can help manage PCOS. Although these diets can initially improve insulin sensitivity and help with weight loss, they might not be suitable or sustainable for everyone with PCOS. To create a customized diet plan that fits your needs and health objectives, speak with a healthcare professional or registered dietitian.

Supplements and their potential to manage PCOS symptoms are a common concern. To ensure safety and efficacy, it's important to use supplements under medical supervision. Some supplements, such as inositol, omega-3 fatty acids, and vitamin D, have shown promising results in improving insulin sensitivity and hormone levels in women with PCOS.

MANAGING PCOS-RELATED CRAVINGS AND EMOTIONAL EATING

Managing cravings and emotional eating can be difficult when dealing with PCOS because of the way hormone imbalances and insulin resistance can increase the desire for sugary or high-fat foods. One way to deal with cravings is to learn how to control them and eat balanced meals throughout the day that include healthy fats, protein, and fiber to help stabilize blood sugar levels and lessen the severity of cravings.

Rather than being the result of physical hunger, emotional eating is frequently the result of stress or other emotional triggers. Reducing access to highly processed or trigger foods and keeping healthier snack options readily available can also help break the cycle of emotional eating. Other strategies to deal with stress include developing coping mechanisms such as meditation, exercise, or hobbies.

A better relationship with food can be fostered by incorporating mindful eating practices, which include paying attention to hunger and fullness cues, eating slowly, and savoring every bite. Seeking support from a therapist or counselor who specializes in emotional eating can provide additional tools and strategies for effectively managing these challenges.

ADVICE FOR SOCIAL EVENTS AND EATING OUT

Planning and awareness are key to managing PCOS when dining out. Restaurants that offer healthier options, such as grilled proteins, salads with dressing on the side, and vegetable-based sides, can help you stick to a PCOS-friendly diet. You can also customize meals to meet dietary needs by asking for substitutions or modifications, like steaming instead of frying or sauce on the side.

Bring a dish or snack to share that fits your dietary needs to ensure there's always a healthy option available. Social gatherings often feature foods that may not be compatible with a PCOS-friendly diet, such as desserts, sugary drinks, or processed snacks. Planning by eating a balanced meal or snack before attending can help reduce temptation and stabilize blood sugar levels.

When it comes to eating out or going to social gatherings, it's important to communicate your needs to others. You can advocate for your dietary preferences and explain why certain foods might not be suitable for you because you have PCOS. You can also emphasize the social aspects of the event and the company you have rather than focusing just on the food, which can help lower stress levels and improve overall well-being.

MANAGING DIETARY CHALLENGES ASSOCIATED WITH PCOS

A multifaceted approach is necessary to manage the diet-related challenges that PCOS presents, including insulin resistance, weight management, and hormonal fluctuations. Regular physical activity, such as aerobic exercise and strength training, can help improve insulin sensitivity and support weight management goals.

 It is important to consult with a healthcare provider or a registered dietitian to develop a personalized meal plan that addresses specific PCOS symptoms and goals.

Monitoring portion sizes and engaging in mindful eating practices can further enhance dietary management of PCOS-related challenges. Balancing macronutrients, such as carbohydrates, proteins, and fats, can help stabilize blood sugar levels and manage insulin resistance associated with PCOS. Opting for whole foods over processed foods and sugars can also reduce inflammation and support overall health.

It is crucial to understand that controlling PCOS with diet may need adjusting over time as symptoms and health objectives change. Consistently monitoring symptoms, like irregular menstruation or weight fluctuations, can direct dietary and lifestyle modifications. Seeking support from medical professionals, support groups, or online communities can offer inspiration, drive, and more tools for effectively managing PCOS.

ADVICE FOR GETTING PROFESSIONAL SUPPORT AND ASSISTANCE

To effectively manage PCOS, it is imperative to seek professional assistance and support, particularly regarding dietary interventions. Consulting with a healthcare provider who specializes in PCOS, such as an endocrinologist or gynecologist, can provide individualized treatment options and personalized medical advice.

In addition to providing instruction on nutrition labels, portion sizes, and meal scheduling to enhance metabolic health and hormone balance, a registered dietitian with experience in PCOS nutrition may offer help in creating a balanced meal plan that addresses individual symptoms and health goals.

Participating in online forums, social media groups, or local support groups may offer opportunities to connect with others facing similar challenges and learn from their experiences. Joining a support group or community for women with PCOS can offer emotional support, shared experiences, and useful tips for managing the condition.

A mental health professional can offer strategies for improving self-esteem, building resilience, and enhancing overall well-being alongside dietary and medical treatments. In certain cases, counseling or therapy may be beneficial for addressing emotional challenges related to PCOS, such as body image issues, stress management, or coping with the impact of symptoms on daily life.